smiles from the Clinic

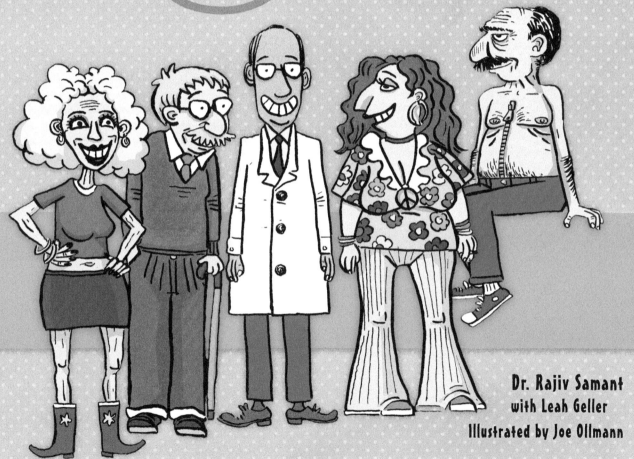

Dr. Rajiv Samant
with Leah Geller
Illustrated by Joe Ollmann

A humorous look at cancer

ACKNOWLEDGEMENTS

They say it takes a village to raise a child, and I completely agree with this sentiment.

I have also discovered that it takes a village, or at least a team of collaborative, like-minded and motivated individuals, to write a book. It would not be possible to personally mention all the friends, family and colleagues who have helped me along the way, but there are clearly some people who need to be recognized.

Firstly, my parents, Jayanti and Hari Samant, who have been incredibly supportive throughout my life journey, with all the bumps and potholes along the way. They gently guided me towards a career in medicine (well, maybe not so gently, since they are immigrant Indian parents after all!) My children, Kristopher, Erin and Keira, who are a constant source of inspiration (and, yes, frustration sometimes!) They have shown me that you must lead by actions, not words. They were the biggest motivators for me – how could I ask them to work hard and be passionate about fulfilling their dreams if I wasn't willing to do the same?

A very special thank you to Sandra Green and her team at Green Communication Design, who have been very eager supporters, giving this book form and function, as well as coming up with our logo. Thank you to Anne DeButte, who was kind enough to share her book writing experience with me and then directed me to Kita Szpak, who made everything so much easier with her words of wisdom and introduced me to Justin Sachs and his fantastic team at Motivational Press.

I also want to acknowledge the help of my friends and colleagues who have provided input and feedback on the stories and pictures – Gabe Duquet, Kate Lochrin, Laval Grimard, Kelly-Anne Baines, Tiffanie Sabourin, Berthe Bourque, Liz Rumball, Hélène Tremblay, Joanne Meng, Jeff Hovey, Carol Stober, Denise Pajot, Jason Pantarotto and Steve Andrusyk.

Finally, a special thanks to all the patients and their family and friends who inspired this book and remind us constantly that, even with a diagnosis of cancer, smiles and humour are essential to move forward in a positive way with our lives...

Design and layout: Green Communication Design inc.

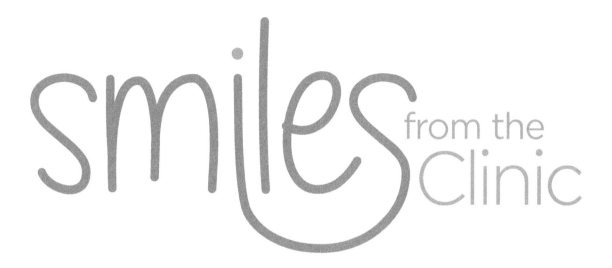

smiles from the Clinic

A humorous look at cancer

 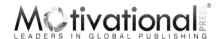
Motivational PRESS®
LEADERS IN GLOBAL PUBLISHING

FOREWORD

You may be wondering why a doctor would attempt to write a (supposedly) humorous book about cancer. Well, I have found that too many people, even other physicians, think that working with cancer patients is very serious business and must be pretty depressing work. However, my experience has been quite the opposite.

The cancer patients with whom I have had the privilege to work with demonstrate humour, smiles and positivity every day. It helps them face their disease, cope with treatment and get on with their lives in a positive and meaningful way. They are definitely among the most grateful people I have ever met, and working with them has made me a happier and better person.

Much of the practice of medicine is about relationships and, as we all know, relationships, at least good relationships, are often filled with humour. Within oncology (the specialty of cancer treatment), just like any other field of medicine, special relationships develop between patients and their physicians, and humour is often involved. That is definitely what I have observed in my clinical practice.

This book is dedicated to cancer patients, as well as their families and friends. All the stories are based on my personal experiences and observations over 25 years of medical practice. Believe me, I am not a comedian or humourist – just ask my kids. I would never be able to make up such funny stories myself.

These stories are meant to show that we all say and do things – often during stressful times – that can make us and those near us laugh and smile. I believe there is humour all around us and we just need to open our eyes, ears and hearts to it.

With this in mind, please enjoy these "Smiles from the Clinic" stories and share them with family, friends and colleagues.

Thank you for your support!

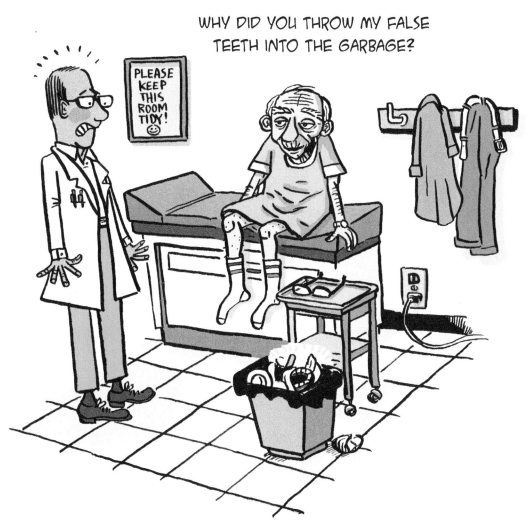

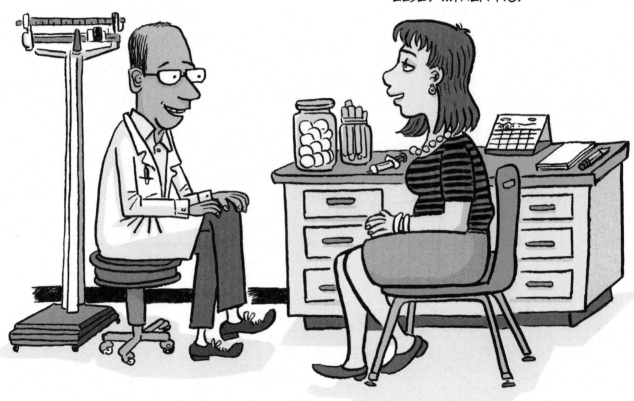

A male patient with prostate cancer in his early seventies asked me, "I have less hair in my armpits and my breasts are swelling. Is that due to hormones?" Then he said with a wink, "I also noticed lately I have to squat to pee, too."

A patient in her early seventies accompanied her husband for his follow-up appointment to the cancer clinic. She was very nervous and unsure, and asked me what could happen if she and her husband took a vacation. I looked at her and said, "Well, you might have some fun."

I was examining a male patient in his sixties and gently thumping him on his back. "Does that hurt?" I asked. "No more than when my wife hits me," he replied.

I saw an 85-year-old woman for endometrial cancer to decide if she might need radiation after her surgery. For the initial consultation, she came with a friend in her sixties who happened to be a former patient of mine. We went through the usual questions and examination, and the plan was for the patient to return in a couple of weeks to make a final decision about radiation.

When I saw her two weeks later I asked, "Where is your friend today?" The patient answered, "I wanted to see you by myself. You see, last time I saw you, I lied. You know when you asked me if I was having sex and I said 'no.' Well, I am having sex and I really like it. You see, my partner is 10 years younger than me, and he tells me that I make him feel like a teenager again. I am embarrassed, but in a good kind of way. Nobody else knows. If my daughter found out, she would have a heart attack. Worst of all, he's not even Jewish!"

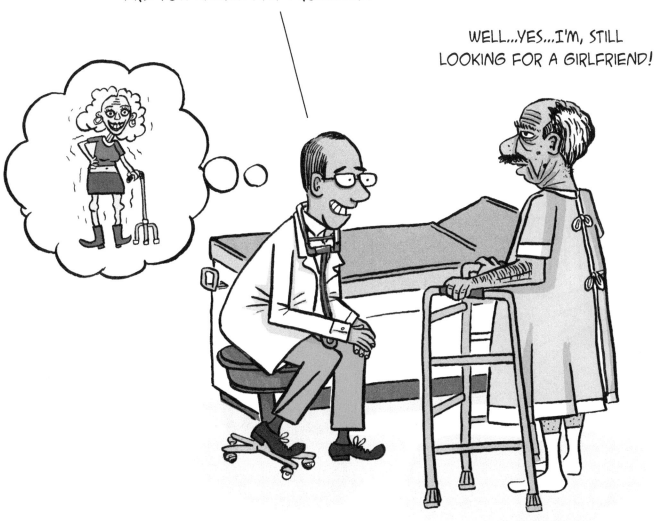

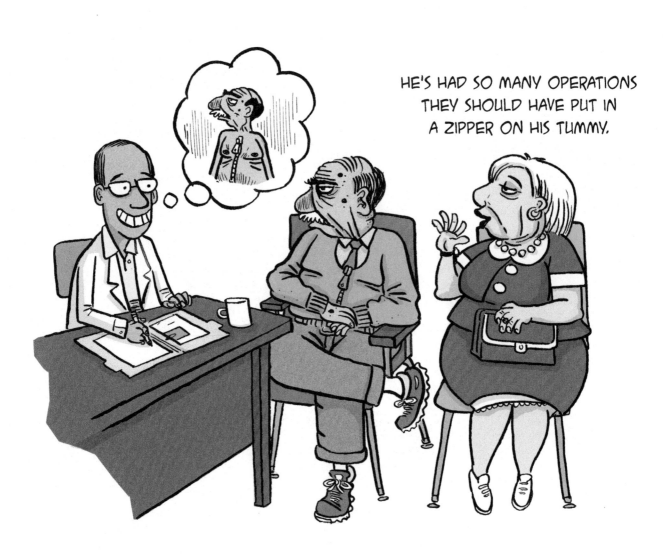

A man in his seventies came to the cancer centre. He was wearing a hearing aid. I asked him if he was sexually active. "Oh yes!" he replied. "I cut the grass regularly and love to go camping."

A man in his fifties was explaining his mother's health situation to me and said, "My mother is blind in one eye and can't see out the other."

A female patient in her sixties came in after completing treatment. I asked her how things were going. "I have a lot of gas since my surgery," she said. "This should make yoga class interesting."

One night at the dinner table, my wife asked our three young children, "Do you know what Daddy does for his job?" "Yes, he is a cancer doctor" they chimed in. "But do you know what kinds of cancer he treats?" she asked. "I treat a lot of prostate cancer," I explained. "What's a prostate?" my 8-year-old boy asked. "It's this organ in men between their rectum and bladder," I replied. "But how do you check it?" the two girls asked. "I use my finger," I said. "Gross! That's weird. I wouldn't do that!" the kids screamed out. "Well, I do wear a glove," I explained. "Ewwwwwww!" said my son.

A few nights later, my son and his friend were walking to the local neighbourhood rink to play ice hockey. My son turned to his friend and said, "Brett, do you know what my dad does for his job? He puts his finger up men's butts to examine something called a prostate." Brett thought for a moment and then said, "Why doesn't he just use a stick instead?"

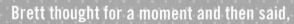
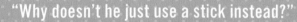

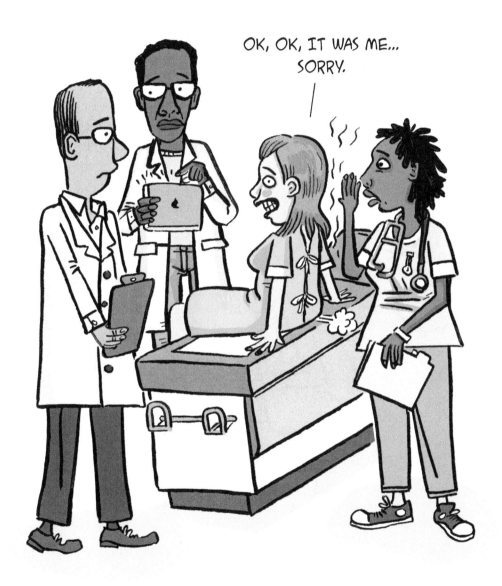

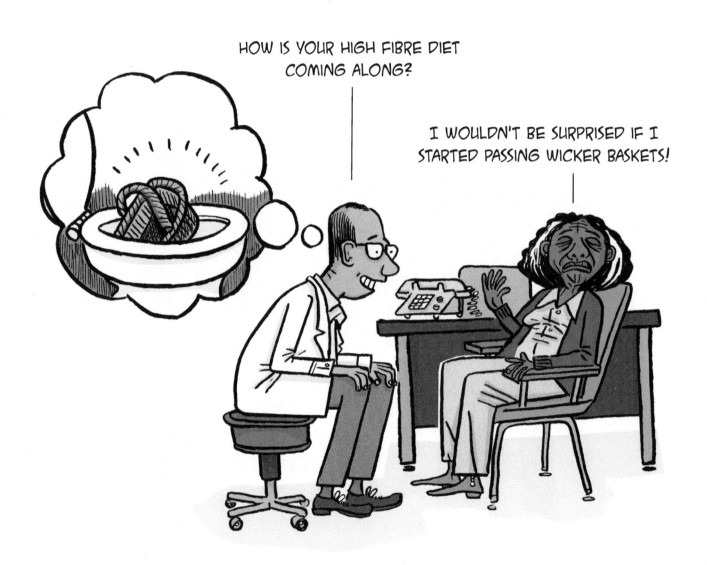

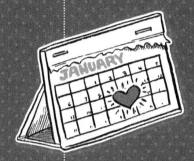

A middle-aged male patient told me about his recent appointment with his kidney specialist. "She was gorgeous," he said. "At the end of my visit, she told me to see her again in six months, and I said, 'Can't you make it sooner?'"

A man in his sixties was asked if his wife had any operations. He answered, "Yes, she's had two hysterectomies."

I asked a patient in her seventies about her sexual history. She replied, "I've been quite active sexually since my husband died."

I once had to perform a gynecologic examination on a retired nun who was recovering from hysterectomy surgery for endometrial cancer. She appeared nervous and anxious, so the nurse and I tried to be as careful and gentle as possible, telling her exactly what we were doing and making sure it was not too uncomfortable for her. After the examination was over, the nun was quite relieved and exclaimed, "Thanks, doctor. That was great!"

Later that evening I told my wife what the nun had said after the examination. My wife calmly turned to me and said "Don't seem so proud. After all, what does she know? She's a nun."

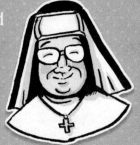

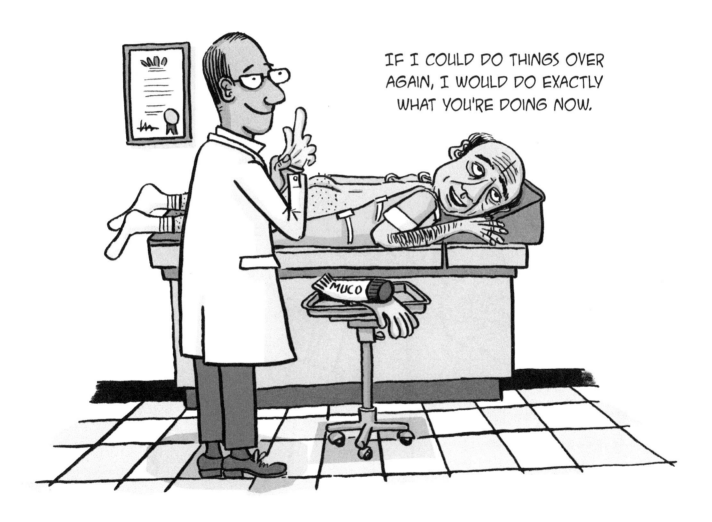

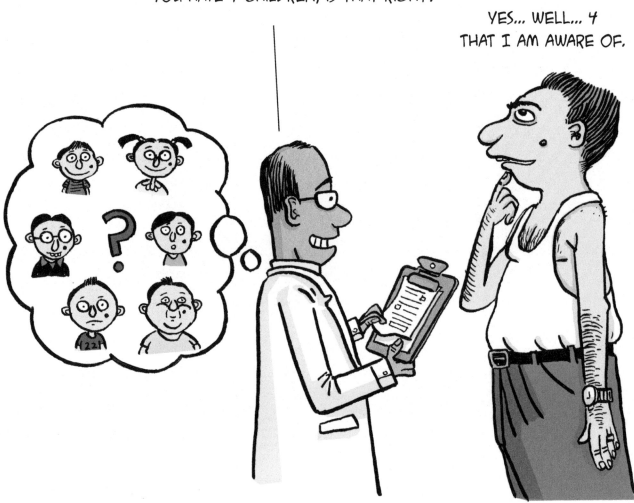

A patient in her seventies was somewhat deaf so we were speaking very loudly in the room. The patient asked whether she needed to keep using the vaginal dilator following treatment. "No," I answered. "You can have sex with your husband instead."

The patient didn't answer and because she was hard of hearing, I repeated even more loudly this time, "I SAID YOU DON'T HAVE TO USE THE DILATOR. YOU CAN HAVE SEX WITH YOUR HUSBAND." She turned to me with a look of disappointment and said, "I know."

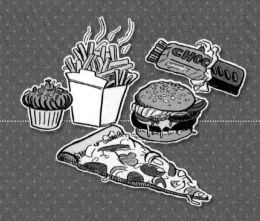

A patient in his seventies who loved telling jokes said to me, "My urologist tells me he will sometimes use two fingers during a digital rectal exam so he can get a second opinion."

A cancer patient in her sixties said to me, "I know I'm gaining weight but I just love to eat. If I'm gonna go, I'm not going to go hungry, that's for sure!"

I asked a patient how many children he had. "We stopped at five," he answered. "Before that, I would ask my wife in bed, 'Do you want to sleep or what?' and she would say, 'What?' But since she started using her hearing aid, she just wants to sleep!"

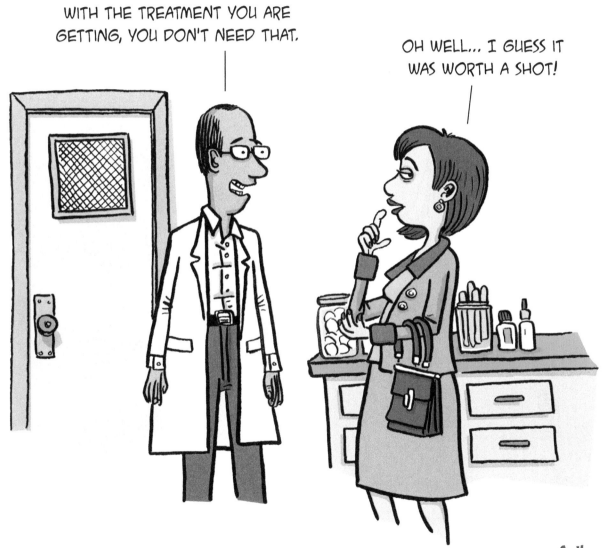

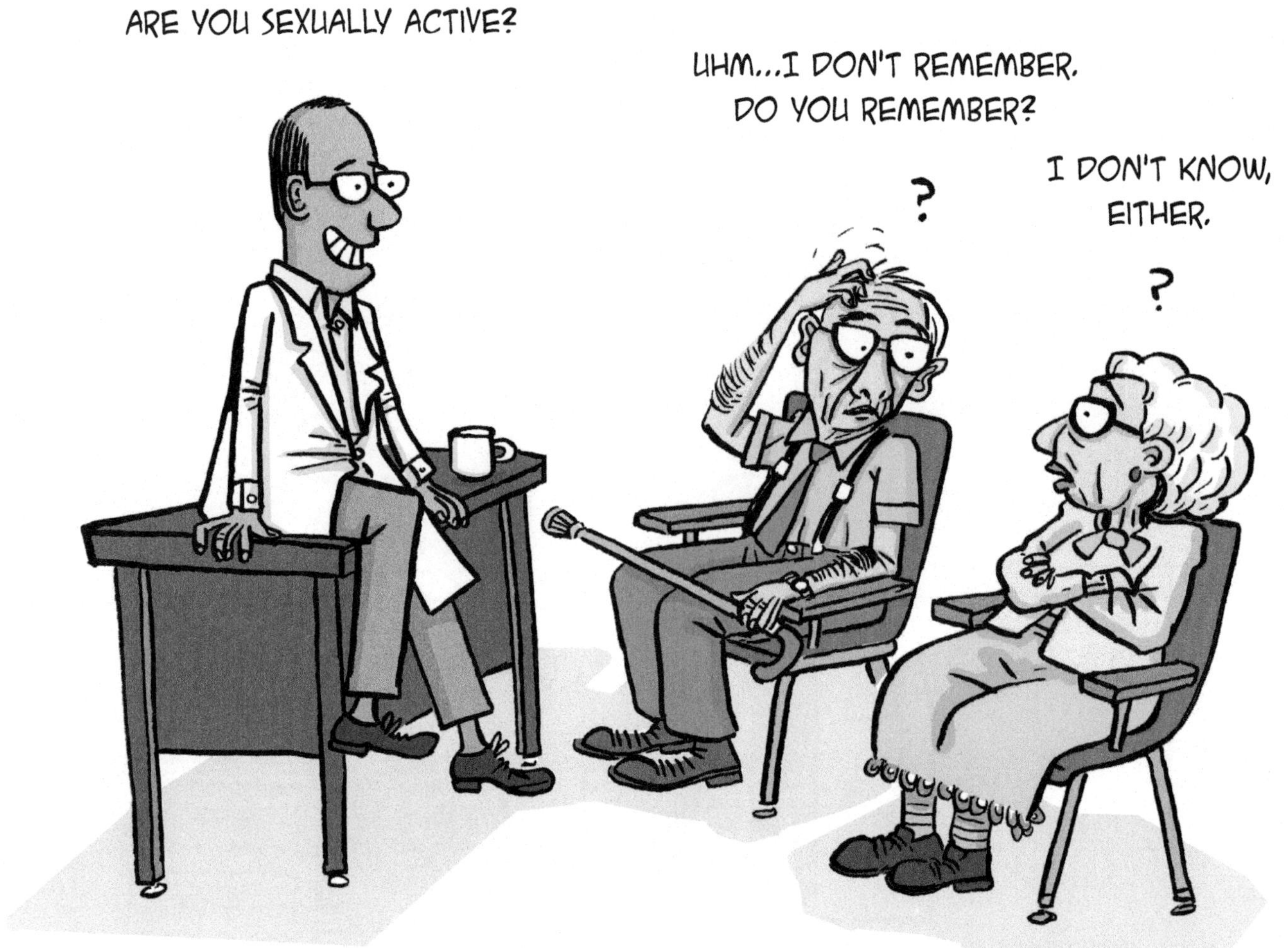
ARE YOU SEXUALLY ACTIVE?
UHM...I DON'T REMEMBER. DO YOU REMEMBER?
?
I DON'T KNOW, EITHER.
?

I saw a very interesting skin cancer patient

in his fifties many years ago. I asked him about his skin cancer on his face, which had been surgically removed.

I started to examine him. His surgical scar was well healed, there was no sign of any cancer and it looked like he did not need any more treatment. Then I noticed something that looked like a large dark raisin on the back of his right ear.

"What's that behind your ear?" I asked. "Have you had something there for some time?" He answered, "Oh, that's my gum. I thought it would be rude to chew it while talking to the doctors so I just hid it there."

An 83-year-old male patient came in who looked 20 years younger than his age. I asked him how he stayed looking so great. "Onions and a good woman," he answered. "At least that's what a 91-year-old friend told me," he added. "But my wife says the woman should come first and the onions second."

I asked a male patient of mine in his sixties if he had any history of cancer in his family. He reflected carefully and responded, "Yes, my aunt, that is, my mother's sister – well, she had prostate cancer."

A patient in her seventies was about to have a gynecologic exam and her husband wasn't sure if he should leave the room. I told him it was up to his wife. She said he could stay. "I'm sure it isn't anything you haven't seen before," I said. "Well, I'm not so sure. It's usually in the dark," he replied.

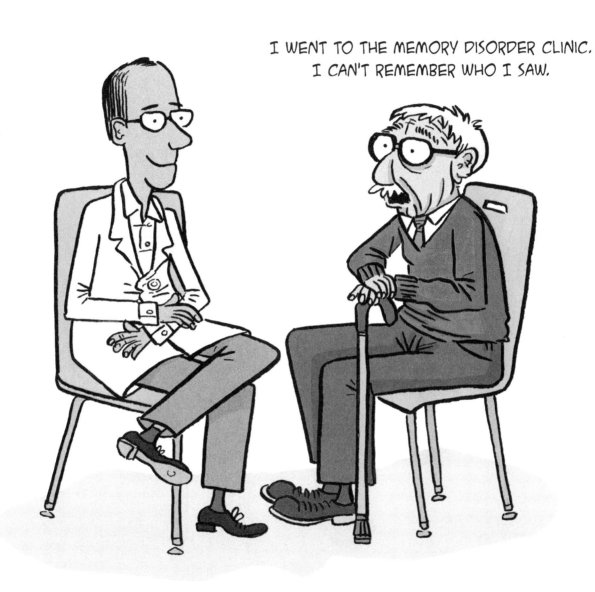

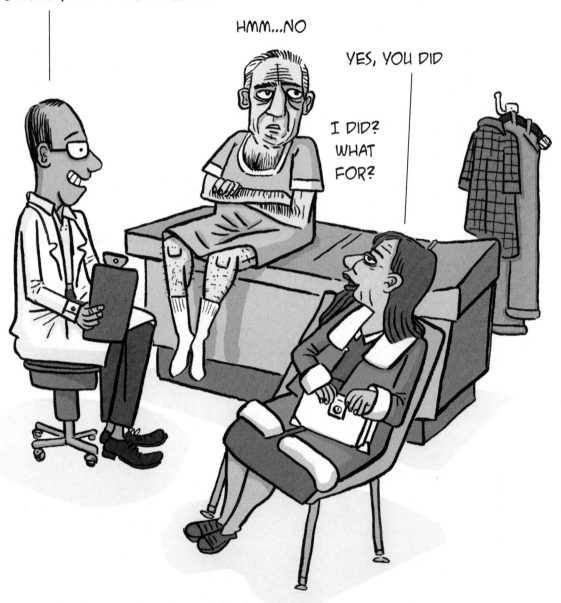

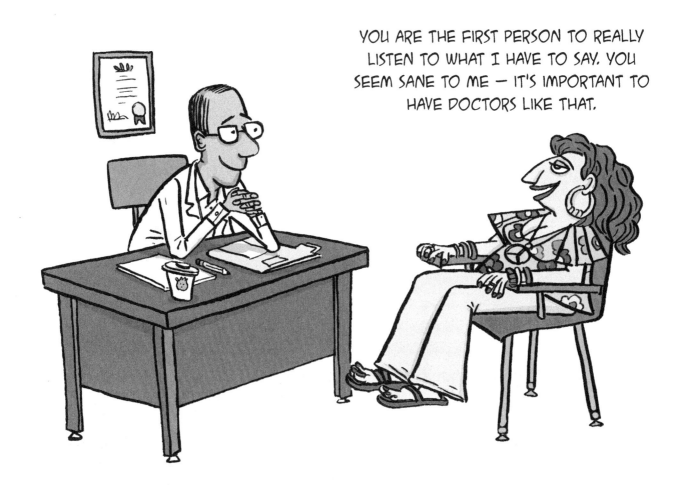

An Italian patient in her late sixties came to see me with another woman about her age. Both were very friendly and had strong Italian accents. The patient introduced me to her friend, and the friend explained that she was going to help translate.

"That is a good idea," I said. "So tell me again, how bad is the pain?"

The friend turned to the patient and said loudly (in English) with a strong accent, "The doctor, he wants to know, how bad is the pain?"

The patient replied (in heavily accented English), "Not bad."

The friend turned towards me and said loudly once again, "She says it not bad."

I chuckled to myself, thinking I could also speak English with an Italian accent if that would help!

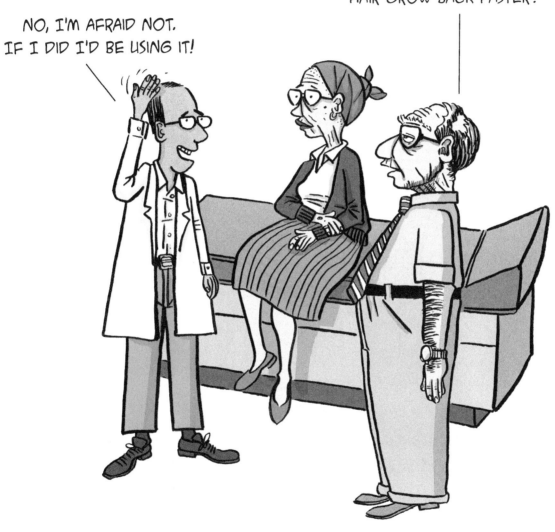

While walking along a busy downtown street,

A YOUNG PATIENT IN HER THIRTIES RECOGNIZED ME AND CAME TO SAY HELLO.

SHE TURNED TO HER GIRLFRIEND AND SAID, "THIS IS THE DOCTOR WHO SAVED MY LIFE, SO I HAVE TO GIVE HIM A HUG."

THEN HER FRIEND RESPONDED, "WELL, IF HE SAVED YOUR LIFE, THEN I HAVE TO GIVE HIM A HUG, TOO."

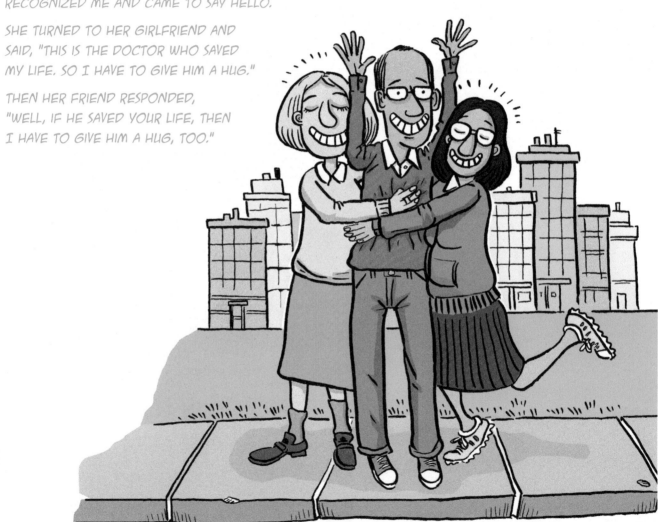

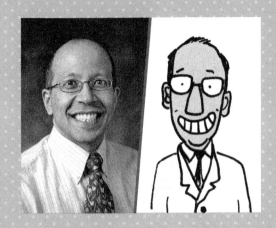

A FEW THOUGHTS FOR REFLECTION

My purpose in writing this book is to highlight an important part of cancer care that I believe is too often ignored – positivity, smiles and humour. What you have read are real-life stories from my work with cancer patients that I believe truly reflect these values. They help me look at life in a positive and hopeful way. After all, this book is really about life, not cancer.

I hope you have found this book entertaining and that it has given you reasons to smile (and even laugh at times!) Whether you are a cancer patient, family member, friend or healthcare professional, remember to focus on the brighter side of life.

My prescription for all of you is a daily dose of smiles and humour – you don't need to go to the pharmacy to fill out this prescription because it is all around you!

Published by Motivational Press, Inc.

1777 Aurora Road

Melbourne, Florida, 32935

www.MotivationalPress.com

Manufactured in the United States of America.

ISBN: 978-1-62865-270-3

CPSIA information can be obtained at www.ICGtesting.com
Printed in the USA
BVOW10s1050250216

437869BV00025B/318/P